Smoothies Against Cancer: Fueling Your Body's Defense

Healthy Eating

Table of Contents

Introduction

Welcome to "Smoothies Against Cancer: Fueling Your Body's Defense"! In this book, we embark on an empowering journey towards harnessing the natural healing powers of wholesome ingredients combined in delicious smoothie recipes. These carefully crafted blends are designed to bolster your body's defenses and support your well-being in the fight against cancer.

Cancer is a formidable adversary, affecting millions of lives worldwide. As we witness the ever-increasing prevalence of this disease, it becomes crucial to equip ourselves with every tool available to combat its impact. One of the most powerful weapons in our arsenal is proper nutrition, and smoothies emerge as an extraordinary ally in our battle against cancer.

Within these pages, you will discover a treasure trove of anti-cancer smoothie recipes, each crafted with a thoughtful combination of ingredients known for their potential in promoting health, strengthening immunity, and aiding in cancer prevention. We have sourced a diverse array of fruits, vegetables, herbs, and superfoods, all rich in vital nutrients and brimming with antioxidants to fuel your body's natural defense mechanisms.

Our mission is to make this journey to better health enjoyable, delicious, and accessible to all. Whether you are seeking ways to enhance your daily nutrition or searching for a supportive approach to complement your existing cancer-fighting strategies, these smoothies offer a delightful and nourishing solution.

Throughout this book, you will find not just recipes, but a deeper understanding of the potent ingredients and their potential impact on your well-being. Each smoothie has been thoughtfully curated to cater to varying taste preferences, dietary needs, and health goals, ensuring that you can find the perfect blend to suit your individual journey.

We encourage you to embrace the transformative power of these smoothies as you take charge of your health and embark on a path of vitality and resilience.

Sip your way to strength, relish the vibrant flavors, and fuel your body's defense against cancer. Remember, each smoothie you create is a step towards nourishment, healing, and reclaiming control over your well-being.

With "Smoothies Against Cancer: Fueling Your Body's Defense," we embark on a shared mission to support and empower one another. Let us blend our way to a healthier, vibrant, and fulfilling life.

Cheers to your health and your journey towards wellness!

Recipe One: Kiwi-Strawberry Sensation

Ingredients:

- 2 ripe kiwis, peeled and chopped
- 1 cup fresh strawberries, hulled and chopped
- 1 ripe banana
- 1 cup plain Greek yogurt (low-fat or non-fat)
- 1 tablespoon honey or a natural sweetener of your choice (adjust for desired sweetness)
- 1/2 cup orange juice (freshly squeezed or store-bought)
- Ice cubes (optional, for a chilled sensation)
- Fresh mint leaves for garnish (optional)

Instructions:

1. Gather Ingredients: Make sure you have all the ingredients ready, including ripe kiwis, fresh strawberries, a ripe banana, plain Greek yogurt, honey or natural

sweetener, orange juice, ice cubes (if desired), and fresh mint leaves for garnish.
2. Prepare Kiwis: Peel the kiwis using a knife or a vegetable peeler. Chop the kiwi flesh into smaller pieces for easier blending.
3. Prepare Strawberries: Wash the strawberries under cold water, remove the green stems (hulls), and chop the strawberries into smaller pieces.
4. Peel and Chop Banana: Peel the ripe banana and chop it into smaller pieces for easier blending.
5. Add Ingredients to Blender: In a blender, add the chopped kiwis, chopped strawberries, chopped banana, and plain Greek yogurt.
6. Sweeten It Up: Add honey or your preferred natural sweetener to the blender. Adjust the amount based on your desired level of sweetness.
7. Splash of Orange: Pour orange juice into the blender. The orange juice will provide a tangy and citrusy flavor to the sensation.
8. Optional: Add Ice Cubes: For an extra refreshing and chilled sensation, you can

add a few ice cubes to the blender before blending.

9. Blend Until Smooth: Secure the blender's lid and start blending the ingredients on low speed. Gradually increase to high speed and blend until all the ingredients are well combined, and the sensation reaches a smooth and creamy consistency.
10. Taste and Adjust: After blending, take a moment to taste the Kiwi-Strawberry Sensation. You can adjust the sweetness or tartness by adding more honey or orange juice if needed.
11. Serve: Pour the Kiwi-Strawberry Sensation into glasses.
12. Optional Garnish: If desired, you can garnish the sensation with a few slices of kiwi, a strawberry slice, or a sprig of fresh mint for an extra touch of visual appeal.
13. Enjoy: Sip and enjoy your delightful and nutrient-packed Kiwi-Strawberry Sensation! This sensational blend is a delightful way to treat yourself to a burst of fruity goodness.

The Kiwi-Strawberry Sensation combines the refreshing and slightly tangy flavor of kiwis with the sweet and juicy taste of strawberries, creating a delightful and flavorful sensation. As you relish each sip of this nutritious and delicious blend, embrace the goodness of kiwi and strawberry in every mouthful. Cheers to the Kiwi-Strawberry Sensation!

Recipe Two: Watermelon-Cucumber Cooler

Ingredients:

- 2 cups fresh watermelon (seedless), chopped
- 1/2 cucumber, peeled and chopped
- 1 tablespoon fresh lime juice
- 1 tablespoon honey or a natural sweetener of your choice (adjust for desired sweetness)
- 1 cup cold water
- Ice cubes (optional, for a chilled cooler)
- Fresh mint leaves for garnish (optional)

Instructions:

1. Gather Ingredients: Make sure you have all the ingredients ready, including fresh seedless watermelon, cucumber, fresh lime juice, honey or natural sweetener, cold water, ice cubes (if desired), and fresh mint leaves for garnish.
2. Prepare Watermelon: Wash the watermelon under cold water, remove the

seeds, and chop the flesh into smaller pieces for easier blending.

3. Prepare Cucumber: Peel the cucumber using a vegetable peeler. Then, chop the cucumber into smaller pieces for easier blending.
4. Add Ingredients to Blender: In a blender, add the chopped watermelon and cucumber.
5. Fresh Lime Juice: Squeeze fresh lime juice into the blender. The lime juice will add a tangy and refreshing flavor to the cooler.
6. Sweeten It Up: Add honey or your preferred natural sweetener to the blender. Adjust the amount based on your desired level of sweetness.
7. Cold Water: Pour cold water into the blender. The water will help to blend the ingredients smoothly and dilute the sweetness to your taste.
8. Optional: Add Ice Cubes: For an extra refreshing and chilled cooler, you can add a few ice cubes to the blender before blending.

9. Blend Until Smooth: Secure the blender's lid and start blending the ingredients on low speed. Gradually increase to high speed and blend until all the ingredients are well combined, and the cooler reaches a smooth and slushy consistency.
10. Taste and Adjust: After blending, take a moment to taste the Watermelon-Cucumber Cooler. You can adjust the sweetness or lime flavor if needed.
11. Serve: Pour the Watermelon-Cucumber Cooler into glasses.
12. Optional Garnish: If desired, you can garnish the cooler with a sprig of fresh mint for an extra touch of visual appeal and added freshness.
13. Enjoy: Sip and enjoy your revitalizing and hydrating Watermelon-Cucumber Cooler! This delightful and thirst-quenching blend is a perfect companion on a hot summer day or any time you crave a cool and refreshing drink.

The Watermelon-Cucumber Cooler combines the juicy sweetness of watermelon with the crispness of cucumber, creating a rejuvenating and hydrating beverage. As you relish each sip of this cooling and flavorful cooler, embrace the revitalization it brings to your body and senses. Cheers to the Watermelon-Cucumber Cooler!

Recipe Three: Blueberry-Beet Boost Smoothie

Ingredients:

- 1 cup blueberries (fresh or frozen)
- 1 medium-sized beet (cooked, peeled, and chopped)
- 1 ripe banana
- 1 tablespoon chia seeds
- 1 cup almond milk (or any plant-based milk of your choice)
- 1 tablespoon honey or a natural sweetener of your choice (adjust for desired sweetness)
- 1/2 teaspoon vanilla extract (optional, for added flavor)
- Ice cubes (optional, for a chilled smoothie)

Instructions:

1. Gather Ingredients: Make sure you have all the ingredients ready, including blueberries, a cooked and peeled beet, a ripe banana, chia seeds, almond milk,

honey or natural sweetener, vanilla extract (if using), and ice cubes (if desired).

2. Prepare Blueberries: If using fresh blueberries, wash them under cold water and remove any stems or leaves.

3. Prepare Beet: Cook the beet until tender (you can boil, steam, or roast it), then peel it and chop it into smaller pieces for easier blending.

4. Peel and Chop Banana: Peel the ripe banana and chop it into smaller pieces for easier blending.

5. Add Ingredients to Blender: In a blender, add the blueberries, cooked and chopped beet, chopped banana, chia seeds, almond milk, honey or natural sweetener, and vanilla extract (if using).

6. Optional: Add Ice Cubes: For a refreshing and cool smoothie, you can add a few ice cubes to the blender before blending.

7. Blend Until Smooth: Secure the blender's lid and start blending the ingredients on low speed. Gradually increase to high speed and blend until all the ingredients are well combined, and the smoothie reaches a creamy and smooth consistency.

8. Taste and Adjust: After blending, take a moment to taste the Blueberry-Beet Boost Smoothie. You can adjust the sweetness or add more honey if needed.
9. Serve: Pour the Blueberry-Beet Boost Smoothie into a glass.
10. Optional Garnish: If desired, you can garnish the smoothie with a few fresh blueberries or a sprinkle of chia seeds for an extra touch of visual appeal.
11. Enjoy: Sip and enjoy your antioxidant-rich and energizing Blueberry-Beet Boost Smoothie! This vibrant and nutritious blend is a great way to kickstart your day or refuel after a workout.

The Blueberry-Beet Boost Smoothie combines the vibrant colors of blueberries and beets with the natural sweetness of banana, offering a nutrient-packed and delicious treat. As you relish the delightful combination of flavors in this healthful smoothie, embrace the nourishment it provides to elevate your well-being. Cheers to the Blueberry-Beet Boost Smoothie!

Recipe Four: Tomato and Basil Refresher

Ingredients:

- 2 large ripe tomatoes
- 1 cup fresh basil leaves
- 1/2 cucumber (peeled and chopped)
- 1 tablespoon fresh lemon juice
- 1 tablespoon extra-virgin olive oil
- 1 garlic clove (optional, for a hint of garlic flavor)
- Salt and pepper to taste
- Ice cubes (optional, for a chilled refresher)
- Fresh basil leaves for garnish (optional)

Instructions:

1. Gather Ingredients: Make sure you have all the ingredients ready, including ripe tomatoes, fresh basil leaves, cucumber, fresh lemon juice, extra-virgin olive oil, garlic clove (if using), salt, pepper, and ice cubes (if desired).
2. Prepare Tomatoes: Wash the tomatoes under cold water and remove the stems.

Chop the tomatoes into smaller pieces for easier blending.

3. Prepare Basil: Wash the fresh basil leaves under cold water and pat them dry with a paper towel.
4. Prepare Cucumber: Peel the cucumber using a vegetable peeler. Then, chop the cucumber into smaller pieces for easier blending.
5. Optional: Add Garlic: If you desire a hint of garlic flavor, you can peel and chop a garlic clove and add it to the blender.
6. Add Ingredients to Blender: In a blender, add the chopped tomatoes, fresh basil leaves, chopped cucumber, fresh lemon juice, extra-virgin olive oil, and garlic (if using).
7. Season with Salt and Pepper: Sprinkle a pinch of salt and pepper into the blender for seasoning.
8. Optional: Add Ice Cubes: For a refreshing and cool refresher, you can add a few ice cubes to the blender before blending.
9. Blend Until Smooth: Secure the blender's lid and start blending the ingredients on low speed. Gradually increase to high

speed and blend until all the ingredients are well combined, and the refresher reaches a smooth and consistent texture.

10. Taste and Adjust: After blending, take a moment to taste the Tomato and Basil Refresher. You can adjust the seasoning or lemon juice to suit your taste preferences.
11. Serve: Pour the Tomato and Basil Refresher into a glass.
12. Optional Garnish: If desired, you can garnish the refresher with a fresh basil leaf or a sprinkle of black pepper for an extra touch of visual appeal.
13. Enjoy: Sip and enjoy your refreshing and savory Tomato and Basil Refresher! This vibrant and herb-infused drink is a perfect way to quench your thirst and awaken your taste buds.

The Tomato and Basil Refresher combines the juicy and tangy flavor of tomatoes with the aromatic essence of fresh basil, resulting in a revitalizing and flavorful drink. As you relish each sip of this garden-fresh refresher, embrace the natural goodness and rejuvenating qualities it

brings to your palate. Cheers to the Tomato and
Basil Refresher!

Recipe Five: Cherry-Almond Bliss Smoothie

Ingredients:

- 1 cup fresh or frozen cherries (pitted)
- 1 ripe banana
- 1 tablespoon almond butter
- 1 cup almond milk (or any plant-based milk of your choice)
- 1 tablespoon honey or a natural sweetener of your choice (adjust for desired sweetness)
- 1/2 teaspoon almond extract (optional, for an extra almond flavor)
- Ice cubes (optional, for a chilled smoothie)

Instructions:

1. Gather Ingredients: Make sure you have all the ingredients ready, including fresh or frozen cherries, a ripe banana, almond butter, almond milk, honey or natural sweetener, almond extract (if using), and ice cubes (if desired).

2. Prepare Cherries: If using fresh cherries, wash them under cold water, remove the stems, and pit them. If using frozen cherries, you can use them directly from the freezer.
3. Peel and Chop Banana: Peel the ripe banana and break it into smaller pieces for easier blending.
4. Add Ingredients to Blender: In a blender, add the pitted cherries, chopped banana, almond butter, almond milk, honey or natural sweetener, and almond extract (if using).
5. Optional: Add Ice Cubes: For a refreshing and cool smoothie, you can add a few ice cubes to the blender before blending.
6. Blend Until Smooth: Secure the blender's lid and start blending the ingredients on low speed. Gradually increase to high speed and blend until all the ingredients are well combined, and the smoothie reaches a creamy and smooth consistency.
7. Taste and Adjust: After blending, take a moment to taste the Cherry-Almond Bliss Smoothie. You can adjust the sweetness

by adding more honey or sweetener if needed.

8. Serve: Pour the Cherry-Almond Bliss Smoothie into a glass.

9. Optional Garnish: If desired, you can garnish the smoothie with a few fresh cherries or a sprinkle of crushed almonds for an extra touch of visual appeal.

10. Enjoy: Sip and enjoy your indulgent and delectable Cherry-Almond Bliss Smoothie! This delightful blend is a wonderful way to satisfy your cravings and treat yourself to a moment of bliss.

The Cherry-Almond Bliss Smoothie combines the rich and sweet flavors of cherries with the nutty goodness of almond butter, creating a creamy and satisfying treat. As you relish the blissful combination of tastes in this luxurious smoothie, embrace the joy it brings to your taste buds and spirit. Cheers to the Cherry-Almond Bliss Smoothie!

Recipe Six: Spinach and Avocado Elixir Smoothie

Ingredients:

- 1 cup fresh spinach leaves
- 1 ripe avocado (peeled and pitted)
- 1 green apple (cored and chopped)
- 1/2 cucumber (peeled and chopped)
- 5-6 fresh mint leaves
- 1 cup coconut water (or regular water)
- Ice cubes (optional, for a chilled smoothie)

Instructions:

1. Gather Ingredients: Make sure you have all the ingredients ready, including fresh spinach leaves, a ripe avocado, a green apple, a cucumber, fresh mint leaves, coconut water (or regular water), and ice cubes (if desired).
2. Prepare Spinach: Wash the fresh spinach leaves under cold water to remove any dirt or impurities.

3. Prepare Avocado: Cut the ripe avocado in half, remove the pit, and scoop out the flesh from the skin. Chop the avocado flesh into smaller pieces for easier blending.
4. Prepare Green Apple: Core the green apple and chop it into smaller pieces.
5. Prepare Cucumber: Peel the cucumber using a vegetable peeler. Then, chop the cucumber into smaller pieces for easier blending.
6. Add Ingredients to Blender: In a blender, add the fresh spinach leaves, chopped avocado, chopped green apple, chopped cucumber, and fresh mint leaves.
7. Pour Coconut Water: Pour coconut water (or regular water) into the blender. The coconut water will provide hydration and a mild sweetness to the smoothie.
8. Optional: Add Ice Cubes: For a refreshing and cool smoothie, you can add a few ice cubes to the blender before blending.
9. Blend Until Smooth: Secure the blender's lid and start blending the ingredients on low speed. Gradually increase to high speed and blend until all the ingredients

are well combined, and the smoothie reaches a creamy and smooth consistency.

10. Taste and Adjust: After blending, take a moment to taste the Spinach and Avocado Elixir Smoothie. You can adjust the sweetness or tanginess by adding more green apple if needed.
11. Serve: Pour the Spinach and Avocado Elixir Smoothie into a glass.
12. Optional Garnish: If desired, you can garnish the smoothie with a sprig of fresh mint or a slice of cucumber for an extra touch of visual appeal.
13. Enjoy: Sip and enjoy your rejuvenating and nutrient-rich Spinach and Avocado Elixir Smoothie! This vibrant and creamy blend is a perfect way to nourish your body with essential vitamins and minerals.

The Spinach and Avocado Elixir Smoothie combines the leafy green goodness of spinach with the creaminess of avocado, creating a luscious and nutritious elixir. As you savor each sip of this refreshing and revitalizing smoothie, embrace the nourishing benefits and vibrant flavors it brings to your day. Cheers to the delightful Spinach and Avocado Elixir Smoothie!

Recipe Seven: Mango-Carrot Sunshine Smoothie

Ingredients:

- 1 ripe mango (peeled, pitted, and chopped)
- 1 large carrot (peeled and chopped)
- 1 cup orange juice (freshly squeezed or store-bought)
- 1/2 cup Greek yogurt (plain, unsweetened; or use plant-based yogurt for a dairy-free option)
- 1 tablespoon fresh lime juice
- Ice cubes (optional, for a chilled smoothie)

Instructions:

1. Gather Ingredients: Make sure you have all the ingredients ready, including a ripe mango, a large carrot, orange juice, Greek yogurt, fresh lime juice, and ice cubes (if desired).
2. Peel and Chop Mango: Peel the ripe mango using a knife or a peeler. Cut the

mango flesh away from the pit and chop it into smaller pieces for easier blending.

3. Prepare Carrot: Peel the large carrot using a vegetable peeler. Then, chop the carrot into smaller pieces for easier blending.
4. Squeeze Fresh Orange Juice: If using freshly squeezed orange juice, extract the juice from ripe oranges. Alternatively, you can use store-bought orange juice.
5. Add Ingredients to Blender: In a blender, add the chopped mango, chopped carrot, orange juice, Greek yogurt, and fresh lime juice.
6. Optional: Add Ice Cubes: For a refreshing and cool smoothie, you can add a few ice cubes to the blender before blending.
7. Blend Until Smooth: Secure the blender's lid and start blending the ingredients on low speed. Gradually increase to high speed and blend until all the ingredients are well combined, and the smoothie reaches a creamy and smooth consistency.
8. Taste and Adjust: After blending, take a moment to taste the Mango-Carrot Sunshine Smoothie. You can adjust the

sweetness or tartness by adding more
mango or lime juice if needed.

9. Serve: Pour the Mango-Carrot Sunshine
    Smoothie into a glass.
10. Optional Garnish: If desired, you can
    garnish the smoothie with a small slice of
    fresh mango or a twist of lime for an extra
    touch of visual appeal.
11. Enjoy: Sip and enjoy your sun-kissed and
    vibrant Mango-Carrot Sunshine
    Smoothie! This tropical and nutritious
    blend is a delightful way to start your day
    or enjoy as a mid-day pick-me-up.

The Mango-Carrot Sunshine Smoothie combines
the tropical sweetness of mango with the vibrant
orange hue of carrots, offering a burst of
sunshine in each sip. As you relish the delightful
combination of flavors in this energizing
smoothie, embrace the nourishment it provides
to brighten your day. Cheers to the sunny
Mango-Carrot Sunshine Smoothie!

Recipe Eight: Pineapple-Turmeric Twist Smoothie

Ingredients:

- 1 cup pineapple chunks
- 1 teaspoon fresh turmeric root (or ½ teaspoon ground turmeric)
- 1 large carrot (peeled and chopped)
- 1 teaspoon fresh ginger
- 1 cup coconut water
- 1 tablespoon fresh lime juice
- Ice cubes (optional, for a chilled smoothie)

Instructions:

1. Gather Ingredients: Make sure you have all the ingredients ready, including pineapple chunks, fresh turmeric root, a large carrot, fresh ginger, coconut water, fresh lime juice, and ice cubes (if desired).
2. Peel and Chop Carrot: Peel the large carrot using a vegetable peeler. Then, chop the carrot into smaller pieces for easier blending.

3. Prepare Pineapple: If using fresh pineapple, peel the pineapple, remove the core, and cut the flesh into chunks. If using frozen pineapple, you can use it directly from the freezer.
4. Peel and Chop Ginger: Peel the fresh ginger and chop it into smaller pieces for easier blending.
5. Add Ingredients to Blender: In a blender, add the pineapple chunks, fresh turmeric root (or ground turmeric), chopped carrot, chopped ginger, and coconut water.
6. Fresh Lime Juice: Squeeze fresh lime juice into the blender. The lime juice will add a tangy and citrusy flavor to the smoothie.
7. Optional: Add Ice Cubes: For a refreshing and cool smoothie, you can add a few ice cubes to the blender before blending.
8. Blend Until Smooth: Secure the blender's lid and start blending the ingredients on low speed. Gradually increase to high speed and blend until all the ingredients are well combined, and the smoothie reaches a creamy and smooth consistency.

9. Taste and Adjust: After blending, take a
   moment to taste the Pineapple-Turmeric
   Twist Smoothie. You can adjust the
   sweetness or tanginess by adding more
   pineapple or lime juice if needed.
10. Serve: Pour the Pineapple-Turmeric Twist
    Smoothie into a glass.
11. Optional Garnish: If desired, you can
    garnish the smoothie with a small slice of
    fresh pineapple or a sprinkle of ground
    turmeric for an extra touch of visual
    appeal.
12. Enjoy: Sip and enjoy your invigorating
    and tropical Pineapple-Turmeric Twist
    Smoothie! This vibrant and healthful
    blend is a wonderful way to brighten up
    your day and boost your well-being.

The Pineapple-Turmeric Twist Smoothie
combines the tropical sweetness of pineapple
with the warm and earthy flavors of turmeric and
ginger, offering a delightful and refreshing treat.
As you savor the unique combination of flavors
in this sunny smoothie, embrace the nourishing
benefits it brings to your body and soul. Cheers

to the uplifting Pineapple-Turmeric Twist Smoothie!

Recipe Nine: Berry-Kale Powerhouse Smoothie

Ingredients:

- 1 cup mixed berries (blueberries, raspberries, strawberries; fresh or frozen)
- 1 cup baby kale or spinach leaves
- 1 ripe banana
- 1 tablespoon ground flaxseeds
- 1/2 cup Greek yogurt (plain, unsweetened; or use plant-based yogurt for a dairy-free option)
- 1 cup almond milk (or any plant-based milk of your choice)
- 1 tablespoon honey or a natural sweetener of your choice (adjust for desired sweetness)

Instructions:

1. Gather Ingredients: Make sure you have all the ingredients ready, including mixed berries, baby kale or spinach leaves, a ripe banana, ground flaxseeds, Greek yogurt, almond milk, and honey or natural sweetener.

2. Prepare Mixed Berries: If using fresh berries, wash them under cold water and remove any stems or leaves.
3. Add Ingredients to Blender: In a blender, add the mixed berries, baby kale or spinach leaves, ripe banana, ground flaxseeds, Greek yogurt, almond milk, and honey or natural sweetener.
4. Blend Until Smooth: Secure the blender's lid and start blending the ingredients on low speed. Gradually increase to high speed and blend until all the ingredients are well combined, and the smoothie reaches a creamy and smooth consistency.
5. Taste and Adjust: After blending, take a moment to taste the Berry-Kale Powerhouse Smoothie. You can adjust the sweetness by adding more honey or sweetener if needed.
6. Serve: Pour the Berry-Kale Powerhouse Smoothie into a glass.
7. Optional Garnish: If desired, you can garnish the smoothie with a few fresh berries or a sprinkle of ground flaxseeds for an extra touch of visual appeal.

8. Enjoy: Sip and enjoy your nutrient-packed and flavorful Berry-Kale Powerhouse Smoothie! This vibrant and wholesome smoothie is a fantastic way to start your day or recharge after a workout.

The Berry-Kale Powerhouse Smoothie brings together the antioxidant-rich goodness of mixed berries with the nutrient-packed baby kale or spinach, offering a refreshing and nourishing experience in each sip. As you relish the burst of flavors and textures in this wholesome blend, embrace the nourishment it provides to fuel your day. Cheers to the invigorating Berry-Kale Powerhouse Smoothie!

Recipe Ten: Red Grape and Grapefruit Fusion Smoothie

Ingredients:

- 1 cup red grapes
- 1 large grapefruit (peeled and deseeded)
- 1 cup coconut water
- 5-6 fresh mint leaves
- Ice cubes (optional, for a chilled smoothie)

Instructions:

1. Gather Ingredients: Ensure you have all the ingredients ready, including red grapes, a large grapefruit, coconut water, fresh mint leaves, and ice cubes (if desired).
2. Prepare Red Grapes: Wash the red grapes under cold water and remove any stems or debris.
3. Prepare Grapefruit: Peel the grapefruit using a knife or your hands, ensuring all the white pith is removed. Deseed the

grapefruit by carefully removing the seeds.

4. Add Ingredients to Blender: In a blender, add the red grapes and the peeled and deseeded grapefruit.
5. Fresh Mint: Add fresh mint leaves to the blender. Mint will add a refreshing and zesty flavor to the smoothie.
6. Pour Coconut Water: Pour coconut water into the blender. The coconut water will provide hydration and a mild sweetness to the smoothie.
7. Optional: Add Ice Cubes: For a refreshing and cool smoothie, you can add a few ice cubes to the blender before blending.
8. Blend Until Smooth: Secure the blender's lid and start blending the ingredients on low speed. Gradually increase to high speed and blend until all the ingredients are well combined, and the smoothie reaches a creamy and smooth consistency.
9. Taste and Adjust: After blending, take a moment to taste the Red Grape and Grapefruit Fusion Smoothie. You can adjust the sweetness or tanginess by

adding more grapes or grapefruit if needed.

10. Serve: Pour the Red Grape and Grapefruit Fusion Smoothie into a glass.

11. Optional Garnish: If desired, you can garnish the smoothie with a sprig of fresh mint or a slice of grapefruit for an extra touch of visual appeal.

12. Enjoy: Sip and enjoy your refreshing and tangy Red Grape and Grapefruit Fusion Smoothie! This vibrant and vitamin-rich smoothie is a wonderful way to quench your thirst and boost your energy.

The Red Grape and Grapefruit Fusion Smoothie combines the natural sweetness of red grapes with the tangy and zesty flavor of grapefruit, resulting in a delightful and refreshing drink. As you relish each sip of this fruity fusion, embrace the nourishing benefits and invigorating taste of this antioxidant-rich blend. Cheers to the vibrant Red Grape and Grapefruit Fusion Smoothie!

Recipe Eleven: Antioxidant Boost Smoothie

Ingredients:

- 1 tablespoon acai berries (frozen puree or powder)
- 1 cup mixed berries (blueberries, raspberries, strawberries; fresh or frozen)
- 1 tablespoon chia seeds
- 1 cup baby spinach or kale leaves
- 1/2 cup Greek yogurt (plain, unsweetened; or use plant-based yogurt for a dairy-free option)
- 1 tablespoon honey or a natural sweetener of your choice (adjust for desired sweetness)
- 1 cup almond milk (or any plant-based milk of your choice)

Instructions:

1. Gather Ingredients: Make sure you have all the ingredients ready, including acai berries (frozen puree or powder), mixed berries, chia seeds, baby spinach or kale

leaves, Greek yogurt, honey or natural sweetener, and almond milk.

2. Soak Chia Seeds: If using chia seeds, you can soak them in water or almond milk for a few minutes before blending. This helps them to become gel-like and easier to blend.

3. Add Ingredients to Blender: In a blender, add the acai berries, mixed berries, soaked chia seeds, baby spinach or kale leaves, Greek yogurt, honey or natural sweetener, and almond milk.

4. Blend Until Smooth: Secure the blender's lid and start blending the ingredients on low speed. Gradually increase to high speed and blend until all the ingredients are well combined, and the smoothie reaches a creamy and smooth consistency.

5. Taste and Adjust: After blending, take a moment to taste the Antioxidant Boost Smoothie. You can adjust the sweetness by adding more honey or sweetener if needed.

6. Serve: Pour the Antioxidant Boost Smoothie into a glass.

7. Optional Garnish: If desired, you can garnish the smoothie with a sprinkle of chia seeds or a few fresh berries for an extra touch of visual appeal.
8. Enjoy: Sip and enjoy your antioxidant-rich and nutritious Antioxidant Boost Smoothie! This vibrant and flavorful smoothie is a fantastic way to start your day or recharge your energy levels.

The Antioxidant Boost Smoothie brings together a powerhouse of antioxidant-rich ingredients, including acai berries, mixed berries, and leafy greens, offering a burst of nutrition in each sip. As you savor this delightful blend, relish the natural sweetness and healthful benefits of these superfood ingredients. Cheers to the refreshing Antioxidant Boost Smoothie!

Recipe Twelve: Cruciferous Green Machine Smoothie

Ingredients:

- 1 cup broccoli florets
- 1 cup cauliflower florets
- 1 cup baby spinach or kale leaves
- 1 green apple (cored and chopped)
- 1 ripe pear (cored and chopped)
- 1/2 cucumber (peeled and chopped)
- 5-6 fresh mint leaves
- 1 cup coconut water (or regular water)
- Ice cubes (optional, for a chilled smoothie)

Instructions:

1. Gather Ingredients: Make sure you have all the ingredients ready, including broccoli florets, cauliflower florets, baby spinach or kale leaves, a green apple, a ripe pear, a cucumber, fresh mint leaves, coconut water (or regular water), and ice cubes (if desired).

2. Prepare Vegetables and Fruits: Wash all
    the vegetables and fruits under cold water.
    Chop the broccoli and cauliflower florets
    into smaller pieces for easier blending.
    Core and chop the green apple and ripe
    pear. Peel the cucumber and chop it as
    well.
3. Add Ingredients to Blender: In a blender,
    add the chopped broccoli florets,
    cauliflower florets, baby spinach or kale
    leaves, chopped green apple, chopped ripe
    pear, chopped cucumber, and fresh mint
    leaves.
4. Pour Coconut Water: Pour coconut water
    (or regular water) into the blender. The
    coconut water will provide hydration and
    a mild sweetness to the smoothie.
5. Optional: Add Ice Cubes: If you prefer a
    chilled smoothie, you can add a few ice
    cubes to the blender before blending.
6. Blend Until Smooth: Secure the blender's
    lid and start blending the ingredients on
    low speed. Gradually increase to high
    speed and blend until all the ingredients
    are well combined, and the smoothie
    reaches a creamy and smooth consistency.

7. Taste and Adjust: After blending, take a moment to taste the Cruciferous Green Machine Smoothie. You can adjust the flavors by adding more apple or pear for sweetness or more cucumber for freshness.
8. Serve: Pour the Cruciferous Green Machine Smoothie into a glass.
9. Optional Garnish: If desired, you can garnish the smoothie with a small sprig of fresh mint or a cucumber slice for an extra touch of visual appeal.
10. Enjoy: Sip and enjoy your revitalizing and nutrient-packed Cruciferous Green Machine Smoothie! This green powerhouse smoothie is a great way to nourish your body with essential vitamins and minerals.

The Cruciferous Green Machine Smoothie combines the nutritional power of cruciferous vegetables with the refreshing sweetness of fruits and the invigorating freshness of mint. As you savor each sip of this green elixir, embrace the healthful benefits of this nutrient-rich blend.

Cheers to the vibrant Cruciferous Green Machine Smoothie!

Recipe Thirteen: Citrus-Carrot Glow Smoothie

Ingredients:

- 1 cup freshly squeezed orange juice
- 1 large carrot (peeled and chopped)
- 1 cup mango chunks (fresh or frozen)
- 1/2 cup Greek yogurt (plain, unsweetened; or use plant-based yogurt for a dairy-free option)
- 1 tablespoon fresh lemon juice
- 1 teaspoon fresh ginger (optional, for an extra kick)
- Ice cubes (optional, for a chilled smoothie)
- Fresh mint leaves for garnish (optional)

Instructions:

1. Gather Ingredients: Ensure you have all the ingredients ready, including freshly squeezed orange juice, a large carrot, mango chunks, Greek yogurt, fresh lemon juice, fresh ginger (if using), ice cubes (if desired), and fresh mint leaves for garnish.

2. Peel and Chop Carrot: Peel the large carrot using a vegetable peeler. Then, chop the carrot into smaller pieces for easier blending.

3. Prepare Mango: If using fresh mango, peel the mango, remove the seed, and cut the flesh into chunks. If using frozen mango, you can use it directly from the freezer.

4. Add Ingredients to Blender: In a blender, add the freshly squeezed orange juice, chopped carrot, mango chunks, and Greek yogurt.

5. Add Fresh Lemon Juice: Squeeze fresh lemon juice into the blender. The lemon juice will add a tangy and citrusy flavor to the smoothie.

6. Optional: Add Fresh Ginger: If you desire an extra kick of spiciness, add fresh ginger to the blender. Peel the ginger and chop it before adding.

7. Optional: Add Ice Cubes: For a refreshing and cool smoothie, you can add a few ice cubes to the blender before blending.

8. Blend Until Smooth: Secure the blender's lid and start blending the ingredients on

low speed. Gradually increase to high speed and blend until all the ingredients are well combined, and the smoothie reaches a creamy and smooth consistency.

9. Taste and Adjust: After blending, take a moment to taste the Citrus-Carrot Glow Smoothie. You can adjust the sweetness or tartness by adding more orange juice or lemon juice if needed.

10. Serve: Pour the Citrus-Carrot Glow Smoothie into a glass.

11. Optional Garnish: If desired, you can garnish the smoothie with a few fresh mint leaves for an extra touch of freshness and visual appeal.

12. Enjoy: Sip and enjoy your revitalizing and nutritious Citrus-Carrot Glow Smoothie! This bright and vitamin-rich smoothie is a perfect way to start your day or boost your energy levels.

The Citrus-Carrot Glow Smoothie not only brings a radiant hue but also combines the natural sweetness of oranges and mangoes with the wholesome goodness of carrots. Savor the invigorating taste and the nourishing blend of citrus and carrot, as you embrace the glow this smoothie brings to your day. Cheers to the refreshing Citrus-Carrot Glow Smoothie!

Recipe Fourteen: Green Tea and Berry Smoothie

Ingredients:

- 1 cup cooled green tea (brewed and chilled)
- 1 cup mixed berries (blueberries, strawberries, raspberries; fresh or frozen)
- 1 cup baby spinach or kale leaves
- 1/2 cup Greek yogurt (plain, unsweetened; or use plant-based yogurt for a dairy-free option)
- 1 tablespoon honey or a natural sweetener of your choice (optional, adjust for desired sweetness)

Instructions:

1. Prepare Green Tea: Brew a cup of green tea using a green tea bag or loose green tea leaves. Let it steep for 3-4 minutes and then let it cool down to room temperature. Once the tea is cooled, you can refrigerate it until it's chilled or add some ice cubes to speed up the cooling process.

2. Gather Ingredients: Ensure you have all the ingredients ready, including the mixed berries, baby spinach or kale, Greek yogurt, and honey or natural sweetener.
3. Blend the Smoothie: In a blender, add the cooled green tea, mixed berries, baby spinach or kale leaves, and Greek yogurt. If you prefer a sweeter smoothie, you can add honey or any natural sweetener of your choice at this stage.
4. Blend Until Smooth: Start blending the ingredients on low speed and gradually increase to high speed. Blend until all the ingredients are well combined, and the smoothie reaches a creamy and smooth consistency.
5. Taste and Adjust: Take a small taste of the smoothie and adjust sweetness if needed by adding more honey or sweetener.
6. Serve: Pour the Green Tea and Berry Smoothie into glasses.
7. Optional Garnish: If desired, you can garnish the smoothie with a few fresh berries or a sprinkle of chia seeds.
8. Enjoy: Sip and enjoy your delicious and nutritious Green Tea and Berry Smoothie!

This refreshing and antioxidant-rich smoothie is a delightful addition to your healthy lifestyle.

The Green Tea and Berry Smoothie not only provides a refreshing and delightful taste but also offers the combined goodness of green tea antioxidants and the nutritional power of berries and leafy greens. As you relish each sip of this vibrant smoothie, bask in the health-boosting properties of these ingredients. Cheers to your journey towards a nourished and revitalized self with the Green Tea and Berry Smoothie!

Recipe Fifteen: Turmeric and Ginger Delight Smoothie

Ingredients:

- 1 cup almond milk (or any plant-based milk of your choice)
- 1 teaspoon fresh turmeric root (or ½ teaspoon ground turmeric)
- 1 teaspoon fresh ginger
- 1 ripe banana
- 1 cup pineapple or mango chunks (fresh or frozen)
- A pinch of black pepper (to enhance the absorption of turmeric)
- A dash of ground cinnamon
- 1 tablespoon ground flaxseeds (optional, for added nutrition and texture)

Instructions:

1. Gather Ingredients: Make sure you have all the ingredients ready, including almond milk, fresh turmeric root, fresh ginger, ripe banana, pineapple or mango

chunks, black pepper, ground cinnamon, and ground flaxseeds.

2. Peel and Chop Turmeric and Ginger: Peel the fresh turmeric root using a spoon or a peeler, and then finely chop it. Peel the fresh ginger and chop it as well. If using ground turmeric and ginger, skip this step.

3. Prepare Fruits: Peel the ripe banana and break it into smaller pieces. If using fresh pineapple or mango, peel and cut them into chunks. If using frozen fruits, you can use them directly from the freezer.

4. Add Ingredients to Blender: In a blender, add the almond milk, chopped turmeric, chopped ginger, ripe banana, and pineapple or mango chunks.

5. Add Black Pepper and Cinnamon: Sprinkle a pinch of black pepper and a dash of ground cinnamon into the blender. Black pepper helps to enhance the absorption of turmeric's beneficial compounds.

6. Optional: Add Flaxseeds: If you wish to include ground flaxseeds for added nutrition and texture, add them to the blender as well.

7. Blend Until Smooth: Secure the blender's lid and start blending the ingredients on low speed. Gradually increase to high speed and blend until all the ingredients are well combined, and the smoothie reaches a creamy and smooth consistency.

8. Taste and Adjust: After blending, take a moment to taste the Turmeric and Ginger Delight Smoothie. You can adjust the flavors by adding more turmeric, ginger, or sweetener if desired.

9. Serve: Pour the Turmeric and Ginger Delight Smoothie into a glass.

10. Optional Garnish: You can garnish the smoothie with a sprinkle of ground cinnamon or a small slice of fresh turmeric for an extra touch of visual appeal.

11. Enjoy: Savor each sip of this vibrant and invigorating Turmeric and Ginger Delight Smoothie! Embrace the warmth of turmeric and the spiciness of ginger as you nourish your body with this healthful concoction.

The Turmeric and Ginger Delight Smoothie not only offers a delightful fusion of flavors but also provides potential health benefits from the anti-inflammatory and antioxidant properties of turmeric and ginger. Relish this smoothie as a nutritious addition to your daily routine and embrace the goodness it brings to your well-being. Cheers to the joy of sipping on the Turmeric and Ginger Delight Smoothie!